Franz Guenter Leicht

Synergies in Healthcare Sector

franzguenter-leicht.info

Publisher: **Leicht Franz Guenter,** 94 Pages, b/w.

To acquire e.g. via www.lulu.com **or**
www.amazon.de

Cover design: Franz Guenter Leicht

Press: Lulu Press, Inc.
         3101 Hillsborough Street
         Raleigh, NC 27607
         United States

ISBN: 978-1-326-58392-7

2nd Edition.

Content

Introduction.

This book deals with the synergy between conventional medicine, naturopathy, alternative medicines and alternative therapies as well with the new professions in medical system. This synergy I consider more urgent than ever in this day and age. So this working-out could serve as a template to work jointly on a conception in this issue.

The aim of this working-out is to motivate people in the field of medical system to become familiar with the hidden causes of disease symptoms and specifically with the symptoms of the new time (Part B). On this occasion I appeal to as many people as possible who are seeking help on the one hand and people who are offering help on the other hand to become familiar with these things. This enables them to get better decision support in the treatment of disease symptoms.

Although I am a physicist and I'm from a scientific area that has dealt so far almost exclusively with the tangible and experienceable things (the physical), I came to the conclusion that we need to go beyond the coarse Material in this issue. This follows clearly from the fact that even the physics demands the existence of dark matter and dark energy. It has even been determined by the physics, how the proportionate share is: Matter about 4%, dark matter about 22% and dark energy about 74%. The term "dark" means, that we have to do with things that are not visible or directly observable with physical measurements. Dark matter and dark energy therefore are understood as the unseen or the invisible, which outweighs with its share of 94% by far the visible matter.

Due to this proportionality it must be concluded that this invisible area has no insignificant influence on visible matter. If we further assume that there is the spiritual that is located above all it is close to say that the Material could be an exclusive product of the spiritual. That this is probably so, it is discussed in detail on my website www.franzguenter-leicht.info.

Accordingly, if the spiritual is the sole cause of the Material, all things that we are calling health, disease, convalescence and disease (as process) could be pure manifestations of spirit. **Therefore we can ask why there is health and disease.** The condition of the body would be something like a measure (scale) or guidance that tells us how strong we are aware of our true self and how much we live a life that corresponds to our true nature as spiritual beings. We can quasi move away from our true nature what is perceivable as disease process or we can move towards to our true nature what is perceivable as convalescence process.

The path to health would thus be described in roughly words as follows: **The path would be to try to live in a way that it corresponds to our true nature.** We do this by opening ourselves for love, freedom and joy and by opening our limits. This we do by listening to inner impulses, by following them as well by reflecting on our soul plan and by always trying to live our life according to this plan. Then diseases and problems gradually give way almost automatically. Then we will intuitively avoid things that would get us in trouble, and do things that facilitate, enrich and delight increasingly our lives. Likewise, we will more and more succeed with time, to do the right thing at the right time in the right place and to be on the right place.

On this path we will get more confident and gain more and more strength. At the end of this path, nothing will be impossible for us. Then we will wholeheartedly pursue our true destiny here on earth. And there it will no longer be necessary to learn through disease or be guided on the way by disease. Because then, body symptoms whatsoever don't make sense anymore as guidance. They are/were only there just because to put ourselves in internal dynamics until we have found to our determination/ to ourselves.

Of course I can't come up here with a panacea, because there is an individual path/ plan of salvation for every human being. That is why it is so important that everyone has to listen to his inner impulses and to follow his own soul plan. The good news is that we have no more to think complicated. Everything reduces to our inner wisdom and inner knowledge which is omniscient and unlimited and which means true freedom.

If the linking to the original knowledge and to the great-matrix (blueprint) has absolutely taken place at the end, then we are aware of our true divinity. This awareness enables us to become conscious creators and allows us to realize our true task here on earth.

We also live in an age of enlightenment. It will be discussed, that the conventional medicine still has a need for education in modern symptoms, about which it will be talked. **In this respect, I appeal also to the representatives of conventional medicine, to familiarize with the processes of subtle energy body and the so-called Light Body symptoms.** It needs the synergy of all disciplines in the medical and healing system, which is also discussed on my website (see sources).

Basic points for a possible synthesis or synergy.

With this book, I would like to contribute, that the wedge, which was driven between the various disciplines in the medical system, can gradually be removed by an Interdisciplinary Dialogue. In this context I would like to list the following basic points, which could be suitable for achieving this synergy in a practical way.

1. **It is considered that each person has self-healing forces, which he can gradually activate.** Likewise, it is considered that in general every person has a spiritual potential that allows him in principle, to reach the independence of mind to say that every man is the architect of his own fortune. Also every person can principally bring this potential for development. How well this is possible for a certain people, depends in particular on his current mental or spiritual condition. As long as this spiritual potential is still partly hidden or undetected, we are faced with any problems that cause us always to seek help on the outside. Regarding healing, we will then seek assistance

that we find in one or more disciplines in the medical system.

2. **It is considered that each of the various disciplines in the medical system are basically legitimate.** However, at a certain health problem not each of the disciplines will be helpful. Which of the disciplines is best for application depends on the specific health problem on the on hand and on to what therapy or medical treatment the help-seeker has an access.

3. **To find out which therapies or medical treatments would promise best success, the exploration of the respective causes are of course of great importance.** In this book, among others, such possible causes are addressed, which, to my knowledge, the classical medicine has not yet considered or recognized. Among others, these are causes that have something to do with the soul plan of man or with subtle energy flows in the body energy system of man.

4. **Because man is not just the physical body, but also has subtle and spiritual aspects, the aids are not confined to the physical plane.** So, those aids thoroughly make sense that have

influence on the subtle and spiritual levels of people, as it is the case in many healing methods of alternative healing (homeopathy, acupuncture, acupressure, spiritual healing, ...).

5. **It is assumed that the higher the level is, on which it can be influenced, the more it is to penetrate to the true cause, the more powerful will be the healing effect.** The influence on the purely physical level, as it mostly seems to be the case in the classic medicine, causes primarily a symptom treatment, but does not solve the problem from the root. Because everyone has spiritual aspects, an effect can take place on the subtle and/or spiritual level through each of the therapies or medical treatments, regardless of discipline. This is of course the case if an influence is exerted directly at the higher levels. This could also be the case if the doctor gives the patient a good feeling, if he builds a sympathy with him or if he encourages him. This may also be the case if the faith of patients is correspondingly large in the effect of treatment. It is e.g. demonstrated that patients had just experienced a recovery when a surgery was simulated to them (pseudo-operation). So, in a report of the University in

Heidelberg (Ruprecht-Karls-Universität Heidelberg) it is to read that after one year the
conditions and quality of life of the pseudo-
operated patients were not worse than those of a
comparable group of patients who underwent an
actual surgery.

6. **Each of the disciplines in medical healthcare
   sector should be a help for self-help.** That is,
   it should be generally followed the intention to
   enable the help-seeker to develop his spiritual
   resources, that he can be aware of his inner
   potential and that he can align his life more and
   more according to his inner impulses.

7. **In total consideration it is to assume that it
   would serve the people best if the different
   disciplines are not set in rivalry to each other
   but if an interdisciplinary dialogue is being
   sought, to make practicable the help for the
   self-help.**

A: Synergy in medical system and the new professions.

Shortcomings of traditional and alternative medicine.

An important basic issue might be: "What helps the people best?" On my view this basic question has to do with the man himself, saying, what he believes that it will help him best. His faith, in turn, has often to do with: This 'what has been proven to date' or 'what is the conventional wisdom' is best. Anyone who believes in conventional medicine assumes that this medicine knows about the causes and effects in the biological processes in the body. The same applies to the scientific medicine and the pharmacist. Most doctors and pharmacists treat their patients according to the knowledge which is gained theoretically and practically by the conventional medicine.

We find that medicine now keeps ready an impressive amount of drugs (medicaments) and boasts with a medicament for almost every complaint and for almost every disease. Therefore, we consider generally a medicament that is approved after examining its pharmaceutical quality and its therapeutic efficacy and safety. Would such a medicament bring the relevant disease for each person to disappear, we would say that the appropriate medication is the cause for the appropriate cure. The same applies to the psychotropic substance. A similar question we also have to the reverse process, to the disease. For example, if a particular virus would evermore cause in all people the corresponding disease, we could say with certainty that this virus is the cause of this or that disease.

We now note, however, that no medicament indicates to 100% its desired effect and that not any virus causes evermore the corresponding disease in everyone. Or it may happen that a patient attains healing, if he gets a certain pill because he believes that an active substance is in it, although there was nothing thereof in it (placebo). In the reverse case a person can experience disease, because he believes that he is bombarded with harmful substances by food or by the environment or because notables as parents, good friend or doctor have made reckless statements, such as: "Because of this or that you have to be sick".

Some people who eat relatively healthy to general health scale, may have to do with more diseases as people who comparatively eat less healthy. Also, it happens time and again that a physician emits a death sentence to the patient after a thorough examination of the diagnosis and that the patient suddenly experiences a healing for inexplicably reasons from the viewpoint of the physician. And so, it seems that we can fix on no clear cause in terms of disease on the one hand and recuperation (convalescence) on the other hand, whether in physical or mental area. Therefore it can be assumed that we are dealing to laws that go beyond the traditional biological understanding. **This could mean that viruses, bacteria, toxins and other external stresses are not the primary cause of diseases. This could also mean that medicaments are not the primary cause of healing and/or that healthy diet is not the primary cause for keeping the body healthy.** Consequently, there seems to be hierarchically superior (deeper) causes which can override certain biological facts that are commonly understood as biological laws.

Certainly, traditional medicine has proved for a relatively long time. On the other hand it has reached its limits, where we must realize that it has not at hand adequate solutions for all suffering, diseases and ailments. Likewise the alternative medicines encounter also limits, for which reason we can come to a similar conclusion. These limits should have to do, inter alia, with the fact that it doesn't always take place a cause-solution. Nevertheless it is to suggest that many of these alternative medicines have, comparatively to classical medicine, a greater potential of influence, because their influence is, owing to their essential nature, settled on higher energy areas in the energy system of man (also applies to animals).

The phenomenon of the placebo effect and its opposite effect, the so-called nocebo effect, leads to conclusions that the development of man and his mental state including his beliefs on these issues could represent a decisive factor.

Diseases or human problems seem to have a significant psychological, mental or spiritual background. This shows the present time more and more. More and more people feel that they come to other truths. More and more people go to the doctor because of certain symptoms, which the doctor no longer can correctly classify (e.g. symptoms because of the influence of the Kundalini energy). Or we realize more and more that the methodology of medication makes people sicker and sicker over time, provided that it acts as pure symptom treatment. Without the causes treatment people seem more and more to learn a certain dependency of the medicaments and seem to experience a kind of symptom displacement due to additional side effects. Currently even the trend seems to prevail, that the current biological understanding in medication and the practical experience from the medication diverge more and more. We have to extend if not to revolutionize completely our current understanding about the true cause of both the recovery (convalescence) and the disease. This applies to both the physical and the psychological realm.

But it is also not the case that we have found in alternative medicine the non plus ultra, so we have to say overall that in this issue nothing engages truly comprehensively (universally valid). So we must say that we have not understood anything and not exhausted all knowledge in this issue.

Currently we are facing a certain paradox.

On one side each of the medical and alternative medicine fields seems to be justified at least in parts. On the other hand none of the medical and alternative medicine fields seems to be the real solution, because none of these treatments performs to the desired success for each person. The greater is the challenge, to get satisfactory responses in physical and emotional range. We human beings should rise to this challenge. For this purpose we can appeal to the latest scientific findings. According to these findings, in the traditional medicine we mainly have to do with symptom treatments and less with the causes-solutions. In the alternative medicines, it may also primarily be a symptom treatment. But depending on the therapist, medical practitioner, doctor (yes, there are also doctors who deal with alternative medicines) or spiritual healer it's being attempted in parallel and partly predominantly to achieve causes-solutions.

How much a cause-solution takes place in that area may inter alia be dependent on the spiritual condition of the person who is seeking help and/ or whether a healing is provided in the soul plan of the help-seeker. Of course, in this case also therapist, medical practitioner, doctor or spiritual healer plays a specific role (see Section "On the subject of spiritual healing and healers"). The cause-solution is therefore desirable because it is emerging more and more that our mental attitudes and beliefs including our inner life concepts are largely, if not exclusively, responsible for any symptoms.

Because there is more energy, which conventional science cannot determine directly but indirectly calls as existent, it is increasingly to suspect that the underlying causes are to be found in these areas. This brings us at the same time in unconscious areas where something like the higher or high self of us is to be assumed that has higher truths, greater insights and greater forces. Therefore, one can easily come to the conclusion that the **symptom treatments**, whatever they may look, **should at most serve as a springboard for finding the true causes**; for nothing else. **Thus, they should be considered temporary.**

Because every man believes in something else, the symptom treatments should initially be guided on the understanding of the respective people. This means that the person should be picked really up where he stands straight, but with the background to get him to come to higher truths, which he has to find in himself and which can only be found in himself. This can for example be done with skillful questions, which let get our clients to think about the possible cause(s) in a sensitive manner.

Thus, in any case, a synergy between the traditional medicine, alternative medicines and alternative therapies is to pursue. This synergy however should always be focused on in terms that the applications are be considered as temporary. This means that a discipline is established parallel or better superordinate to these applications that brings or motivates people who are seeking help to go into their own responsibility by pondering/reflecting their inner truth, their inner healing and their creative powers.

We know that everyone has healing powers and that cure can take place without medicaments and without further action in the outer. The phenomenon of placebo and nocebo as well as the knowledge to the ability to change our lives purposefully (power of thoughts, of emotions, of feelings and visions), are evidence enough to lay emphasis on the self-healing. **Very good approaches to this issue also provides the so-called <u>epigenetics</u>** (see sources).

Epigenetics quasi describes the higher level of genetic regulation. So, for example, the renowned scientist and cell biologist Ph.D. Bruce Lipton has found out that the genes do not really control our organism. According to his findings, the genes are not capable of the stand-alone controlling, although they contain the plan of the organism. For a real control, it takes more than just a plan. It is no different than if planning a house. The architect's plan is only a plan that cannot control or rewrite itself. It is the architect who does or can do this. Bruce Lipton has not only found out an analogous principle in stem cells but also brought forward.

What are stem cells? Such body cells, which can develop into all cell types of the organism, are generally be called as stem cells. **To the experiment:** If stem cells were exposed to a specific environment (information field), it was found that, depending on the environment, the one evolved into muscle cells, the others to bone cells and others again to fat cells. The experiments on stem cells pointed out that the information field of the environment was responsible for the development of the cells. Therefore the gene itself does not determine whether the stem cell should evolve into a muscle, fat or any other cells.

The same applies to the formation of proteins. For example, our body can produce 150000 different proteins. But according to the ancient understanding of biology 150000 genes would be necessary for that. But we only have about 23000 genes. So, the genes cannot really control which are to be formed of the proteins. Again, an information field is necessary for that.

Further investigations revealed that the electromagnetic field of our heart interacts with the DNA. The field of our heart is the strongest field of our body. Thus, for example, the electrical field of the heart (ECG) is up to 100 times stronger than the electric field of the brain (EEG). The magnetic field of the heart is even up to 5000 times stronger than the magnetic field of the brain.

Now, the electromagnetic field emits a signal which passes via the receptors of the cell membrane to the DNA. As a result of these receive-signals, the switching of genes is altered. In consequence the reading of the gene blueprint and thus the protein production is changing. That is to say, the biology of our bodies is changing depending on the receive-signals.

These considerations and other experiments suggested the assumption that we control the genes by our way of life, our beliefs and feelings, though mostly unconsciously. So, our beliefs, convictions and feelings create an information field that is responsible for how the genes are read and which proteins are formed.

If we, for example, are thinking constantly that we are healthy, vital and powerful, the genes are read in a way that we favor the rehabilitation and strengthening of the body or maintain a healthy and vigorous condition of the body. **These new findings have far-reaching consequences because they represent our current understanding on the head.** While we previously have seen ourselves more or less powerless against our body condition or/ and against the outer world, we know now that we are indeed not so powerless. We have our health and our lives in our own hands to a large extent. We are by our thoughts, feelings, visions, fears, beliefs and our inner concepts the architect who is responsible for his genetic plan. Ultimately, we ourselves are responsible for the constitution/ the state of our body. Subsequent section illustrates our power potential at least in terms of our self-healing.

Deeper meaning of the term "medicament".

When I looked for my own Codex (part C) and I came across the "Codex Medicamentarius", I realized that new findings make it necessary to rethink certain things on this issue. This is perhaps more understandable if we look closer at the deeper meaning of the term "medicament". The word "medicament" is composed of the two terms: **"medicus"** and **"mens"** (genitive form: mentis). "Medicus" is the Latin word for doctor and healer, and "mens" is the Latin word for spirit and mind.

So "medicament" means, that the spirit is the actual doctor or healer and that not the material aspect of a pill is equipped with a healing function. We all are living energy. And living energy is never ineffective. Therefore, there is a cause for each symptom or problem of every human being that must be find out. Two people who are in the same environment can be confronted with different symptoms/problems. Specifically, two people can carry in their body the same bacteria or viruses and can still show different symptoms (in the one it emerges a corresponding symptom and in the other not), which suggests that the individual symptom or problem has to do with the individual cause and thus with the individual human. So if someone perceives a specific symptom, the true cause of his symptoms is to look within himself/ in his spiritual condition. In other words, this means that the life-situation of a person always has to do with himself; so it is not really a random coincidence.

Every person has just by his energetic existence an ever-lasting creative power and thus is constantly acting in any way. Realizing this it infers that every human being has self-healing and creative powers, which in principle enable him to be completely independent and free. From these findings phenomena can be derived which are known as placebo and nocebo.

Furthermore, the terms "medicament" and "medium" have the same root word. "Medium" is the Latin word for medium, middle, center. So, through this common root word we can also recognize the path to our healing. It is the path to the center, which means the connection with our inmost essence (the true center).

In summary, over the deeper meaning of the word "medicament" it can be argued that in every man resides an inner healer (the real medicament), who is the really able to heal. This healer has true wisdom that we can make ourselves available by calling over (by invoking) or/and by connecting with it.

Presumably we don't even need to call or ask the inner healer for anything, because his task is none other than to heal. If a petition, then preferably in the form of a prayer of thanks. What matters is to know that he is always in us and always acts in us. This, we can make aware by thinking or speaking of the following over and over again: *"Dear inner healer, nice that you are there and that you act in/ through me. I thank you that you all heal in me, if I only let do your work and if I don't push against your influence by means of my pathological and self-destructive thoughts or feelings. I listen to hear what you are telling me if it requires certain corrections in my pathological thoughts, feelings and behavior. ... "*. Of course each can choose his own words or thoughts.

The aura and the modern symptoms.

Conventional medicine does not teach the energies of the aura and also teaches nothing about the events in the aura. This shortcoming must urgently be compensated, because we are dealing with energetic influences that affect the physical body. The aura, which is a system of several subtle energy bodies of different vibrations, is for most people (still) invisible, but is perceived or felt by more and more people.

Accordingly, there are many findings on this issue although there is still no unified doctrine, which in other respects is not different in the natural sciences. In physics there is still no unified theory. We know about phenomena that do not explain the physics, but which are explainable with the involvement of the invisible (subtle, mental and spiritual area). However, there is now evidence from the Physics to demand outright the existence of the invisible.

The Physics postulates now the existence of dark matter and dark energy. It even has determined how the percentage ratios are: Matter about 4%, dark matter about 22% and dark energy about 74%. Although it does not speak of spirit, but with the requirement of the existence of dark energy it opens the path that could lead us to spirit.

Especially in today's time more and more symptoms emerge on people that cannot explained from the doctors in conventional medicine, what I could identify personally on a client who I had supervised about 3 months in 2011. That woman had, inter alia, repeatedly experienced flashes of light on the body for which there are quite explanations, but traditional medicine does not know (for example symptoms of Kundalini activity). The Kundalini, which is in every human being, is a subtle energy that naturally can have an impact on our physical body. In conjunction with its influence such symptoms can emerge in certain circumstances that so many people can get frightened feelings without that is a real reason to fear there, because of lack knowledge of the real causes.

Given the steady increase of the phenomenon of poorly understood symptoms (in the classical sense), I consider it expedient to address possible causes in this issue. To this topic it can be discussed in a special forum, where own experiences can be exchanged in order to can better understand the mentioned symptoms. I have found personally things that made me suspect that pain can occur in different ways (detailed consideration see part B). On the one hand, a pain may show up if we got an infection or a disease in classical sense or if I hurt my body. Or it can emerge as out of nowhere on the other hand, without I have experienced any injury or disease at the present time. In a particular case, I had about 2-3 weeks pain in the upper body. Sometimes I found it difficult to breathe. It occurred to me the thought that this pain could originate from previous injuries.

It was as if I had been pierced in a previous life of several daggers. If so, this would mean that now something, which I still dragged around with me, was ready to be transformed to light. Perhaps I should say that I perceive Kundalini activities for about 21 years and that during this period various side effects emerged, which, inter alia, have been expressed here and there in the form of temporary pains.

In the case that I got injured or a disease and thereby I feel a pain, it tells me something. This could tell me many things, which we could bring to a common denominator. This denominator could mean that over the pain we should be diverted from our current path, because we would keep us away from the awareness of our true divinity, if we would continue this path. In other words. Over the pain we are forced repeatedly to pause, that we are able to think or feel about ourselves and about the world to get into a mental attitude (mindset) that can evoke our spiritual consciousness and that can bring us at the end into the state of spiritual awareness. In state of spiritual awareness we would have found true fulfillment and therefore we will do nothing that would injure our body or would inflict pain on us or the other.

On the path to our spiritual awareness, we will be faced, to my knowledge, with different pain-phenomena. The one kind of pain is something of a warning sign, which will bring us on the path to ourselves and which will remind us that we have gone really astray. Once we are progressed on our journey of self-discovery so far that we generally are very relaxed, very self-conscious and with great confidence to the day's work or/and to the future, we perhaps will be primarily confronted with symptoms or pains which emerge out of the blue for transformation.

In order we give ourselves to joy, we open ourselves to the external and internal influences, we are increasingly become the observer of our lives and we live our lives in trust, it makes us receptive to higher energies. We live in a time in which intensified external energies (cosmic energy and other energies) and inner energies are flowing. It is the time of the energy work on ourselves, the time of making ourselves reinforced receptive for higher energies but also the time of an enhanced interaction of beings of all kinds, what is generally an act of energetic conjunction and of an energetic moving-together. With this energetic conjunction a harmonic resonance will be built within our energy-body system by which its energy density will be dissolved more and more. While the energy density dissolves a bit, energy is released. The liberated energy in turn dissolves existing energy blockades, old thinking and/or behavior patterns as well brings back memories of past injuries or pains, which may cause short-term symptoms. If this symptoms emerge they come normally one last time in an attenuated form of pain, discomfort, sadness or depression to light, then to disappear forever. Exactly these symptoms can no more really diagnosed in the classical sense.

In general, we need to accept these symptoms or perceived problems with a certain smile and to let them pass us who we are just the observer. Just as they came suddenly out of the blue, they will disappear like out of the blue again, although they may last for about 2-4 weeks or less. Depending on the situation, we also can make use of medicines for the purpose of relief. But this will be a matter quite of a short time, how we can usually observe it. Of course symptoms will still emerge that traditional medicine considers as difficult to cure or even incurable. Such symptoms can be based on deeper things, as we will discuss in part B. Nevertheless, for such symptoms the appropriate person is still faced with the question how it is to deal with that or how he himself would deal with it.

The new professions in the medical system.

The ability of man is a talent that is predisposed (designed) in him as a potential, which he can bring to develop in the course of his life. Aptitudes, talents or abilities are independent of any acquired certificates or titles. This means that these things cannot be transferred from other people. Well, other people can help us in the development, saying, they can promote them in any form. In many cases, people are judged according to their acquired certificates or titles, because it is believed that they can help other people only if they apply any theories or practical things that have somehow practically proven. But we have already shown that probably it's about something else in terms of disease and healing, as to what the conventional medicine teaches us. **Therefore, it needs people who can rise above the conventional medicine and traditional psychotherapy and who have a deeper understanding of how the body, mind and spirit are connected.**

We have now attained a knowledge that has led us more and more to the realization that only a completely different understanding does help us more. It is an intuitive understanding, the understanding with the heart. More and more people seek this knowledge to apply with wisdom. They are also trained, not by people but by an inner teacher or by the spiritual world in accordance with their inner teacher. These people help if they are honest not by making people dependent, but by offering a help for self-help and self-healing. This type of assistance accordingly entails new jobs.

New to these professions is that they act on the energy systems of the human body and the human psyche. The one who provides help then is something like an energetic catalyst for setting in motion the healing process on client or patient if that is ready for it or if the healing is provided in the soul-plan.

In case that two people come together to enter into harmonic resonance, that is, to join together in the spirit, then they allow that energy can flow in their energy systems. This energy is getting free to convert disharmonious energies of certain areas of the human body energy system in harmonious energy, which is always associated with a cure. Only then we can speak of a real healing process.

What have positive wishes, hearty prayers, mental training, spiritual healing, imposition of hands and the like in common? These are energetic actions that affect us and others in the sense that an energetic connection takes place with the above-mentioned accompanying effects. In the type of energetic action there is no limit. The ability of such influences lies in our all natural. No one is exempt. Precisely because in every human being dwells each potential, every person is able to bring for himself to develop that, which makes him healthy and brings him success, if he is not so much blunted in the spirit that it is currently (in this existence) not (any more) possible for him.

If therapist and client join together in the spirit, what for example is the case when a position of trust is set or a certain resonance is established (through sympathy, positive intention, ...), a flow of higher energies takes place in our body energy system. In case, that higher energies pass through us, certain areas of our energy body system can be illuminated, so to speak, that unprocessed memories come to light in any form. This can manifest in the form of sudden pains at certain points in the body, by sadness, depression or by hearty laughter. Such phenomena or symptoms I would interpret as so-called Light Body symptoms. Therapist, healer, life companion and the like should be aware of this phenomena and ready for an aftercare of their clients.

Approach for a concept to get this synergy in a practical way.

The concept could be oriented in a way that it takes into account all stages of spiritual development of a person. Whether we look at a person who goes through all the stages or at many people who are at different stages of spiritual development, it remains conceptually the same. At lower levels it is inevitable that a man eat as healthy as possible, that he eats food of low pollution and/or that he accepts medical aids whatsoever, while at the highest level of his mental development a man could consume deadly poison without that it would harm his body. At the highest level a person would never need a medicament or therapy. He could, if it corresponds to his life plan, even live without food.

Everyone is on a certain intellectual level or in different mental entanglement, as always we want to call this type of state. It is crucial that every human being can change its state and can ultimately reach a level that enables him to overcome any illness, even to overcome death.

Diseases, failures and problems of any kind can be regarded as pure creations that man creates himself or he has created himself. Of course, positive seeming things like health, success, wealth, prosperity and the like can also be regarded as pure creations. Thus, everyone has to answer for everything.

All in all it must be assumed that there is an internal plan for every person who can let remind him (again) at the end that he is divine. With this recollection he is brought to the realization that he is the creator of his own life and that he in reality is dependent on nothing and no one else but on himself. **Only his thoughts, feelings and beliefs determine his life, bearing in mind, that each person also has higher consciousness that shape his life.** The ultimate aim is that man creates a harmony with all his consciousness-parts, if he wants truly to cope with life. He can do this by the fact that he constantly tries to remember what his internal plan (plan soul) is and that he follows his intuition more and more.

In this issue we can split up people roughly into four categories. The man of the first category relies mainly on his mind and on the past experience. Because he's not aware of his spiritual identity and do not know what this really means, his life is geared more on fight, defense, delineation and stress. He sees in the external things a certain power. He might be in a spiritual entanglement of fairly high degree, because he has to realize again and again that his beliefs don't really have consistency because of the many exceptions regarding his understanding. Yesterday he believed to have understood this or that. Today he is also no longer safe and doubt it. He constantly oscillates back and forth between: "I understand, how life works" and "I don't understand the world anymore".

The man of the second category is someone who already begins to question old concepts and old beliefs. That begins to realize that there is more than we can see with the eyes and can find with the physical measurement instruments. He recognizes gradually more and more that he has spiritual powers. Because he does not always see the desired success with his change in thinking, he's still quite strong at doubts. His awaited success therefore still stays partially out, because unconscious beliefs and convictions are still anchored in him which let manifest partially those things which stands in contradiction to his desire.

The man of the third category is able to rise above the many doubts and finds more and more that his life is on the right track. He has reached a self-confidence that does really no more let him shaken. His belief in his spiritual powers and his spiritual guidance has already become a certainty. External influences (radiation, pollutants and toxins) no longer affect his body so strong, because his inner thinking program has quite strongly fixed on stability, flexibility, wholeness, vitality and integrity. He needs not so much to pay attention to healthy diet and can indulge the pleasures always more carefree, without damaging his body.

The man of the fourth category has completely taken away those beliefs that do not match his true divinity. He is now aware of his true divinity and has full access to his higher consciousness parts. He remembers both his true being and his task he has set out to do here on earth. Because he lives his life in perfect harmony with his higher consciousness parts and is fully aware of the power of his thoughts, he cherishes no thoughts anymore which makes his life difficult or unpleasant. On the contrary, he will be at any moment at the right place to think, to say and do the right thing. For such a man deficiency, disease and fights will henceforth belong to the past. Such a person could in certain circumstances consume a deadly poison that does not really hurt him. Whether he does that or something else or he holds himself back to do something like that, it will always be in accordance with his higher consciousness parts. Possibly he has permanently perfected the connection to his great-matrix that his cells can absorb subtle energy for utilizing for food.

According to this view, the rough classification into 4 categories could be very helpful to promote the synergy of classical medicine, alternative medicines and alternative therapies. Because, if we can well estimate a man in this issue we can also well recommend means for help. **Of course a man of the 4th category has successfully reached the end of his therapy.**

Because each person is located in the development, it can be assumed that every human being climbs the categories stage for stage, wherein the fourth stage is the highest (final) stage. Where a person is standing will be pointed out.

The man of the 1st category will mainly take traditional medicine, although that usually treats only symptoms but not searches for the root causes. That man would do well to eat healthy and avoid toxic substances. However, it is at the present time not so simple, to eat healthy and food of low pollution, especially since there is increasingly a lack of nutrients in the food and since the food is always more poisoned and irradiated. It partially lacks of money for quality food or of the time for an own cultivation, etc. The man does not really resolve diseases and bad states of affairs. On the contrary, diseases and bad states of affairs are relocated or even strengthened. So this man is virtually in a vicious circle. But at some point he gets to a point where he can no longer bear his illness or his suffering and he has come at his wits' end. This is the opportunity of rethinking and thus the chance to transform the vicious circle into a virtuous circle. Now, he has the chance and the opportunity to become the man of the category 2, if he really grasps the opportunity.

Man of the second category now begins to question what brings his life to him. He wonders about the meaning of his disease(s) and living conditions, and knows that he causes them at least partially. He pays now more attention to what his body and soul need. In medicine, he now no longer looks so much the panacea and now takes just wisely medication. His attention is now focused on alternative healing. However, he recognizes that even alternative therapies such as acupuncture and homeopathy do not always lead to the desired success. He also realizes that his rethinking does not always lead to desired success, so he still is torn between classical medicine, alternative medicine and mental work. The more he enters the risk of relying on his power of thought, the more secure he's with time, because his unconscious beliefs and old beliefs are losing breeding ground and therefore stand no longer so much in contradiction to his desire. He can see how his life is more and more on the right track. The fact that he can remain steadfast against many doubts and smaller setbacks, he can determine that his faith has become more certainty. His self-confidence is now grown so much that he does make nothing else and no one else responsible for his life but himself. He has climbed the Level 3.

Man of third Category is not yet entirely free from any complaints, but takes only rarely medicaments, whether classical or homoeopathic. In his complaints he sees not even a reason to rethink his life, because his rethinking anyway is already fully under way and he considers anyway to follow his intuition. Where are the complaints coming? By opening ourselves to our soul plan and also to the energies that flow in our energy body system, the remaining unconscious memories, which are characterized by pain and injury, are coming again in an attenuated form to light for being reconciled, purified and transformed. In this way we can let go of the past entirely and also of the related hindering convictions or beliefs. This can be seen practically by the fact that certain symptoms come and go without they hurt us. We let them come and accept them gratefully in the knowledge that they now disappear forever. Now we can let go the related old memories lovingly, if they ever become conscious. Some of the memories do not come by dissolving (reconciliation) into consciousness. A symptom treatment we do only make in exceptional cases for reducing pain. This we will do intuitively correct.

Someday there will be no more unreconciled event from the past which should be brought to light because all unholy thoughts from the past will then be reconciled. Because now no more breeding ground exists for the denial of what we really are, the memory of our true being and our earthly mission (true destiny) can now emerge from the shadows. Now, no more symptoms are coming out of nowhere or would be created at the present time because we are conscious enough, not to create them deliberately. They simply make no more sense. Now we have become the people of the category 4.

The man of the 4th category has successfully reached the end of his therapy and is in harmony with himself. Because his state of mind is perfectly healthy, his body is perfectly healthy, according to the understanding of 'mens sana in corpore sano', in a healthy body, a healthy mind.

Possible measures depending on the category (in brief).

Category 1: medicaments, surgery, healthy diet, tailored food choices (what's good for the body, what not), to avoid pollutants + relaxation therapies (dance, music, game ...) or/and various therapies (Physio therapies, chiropractic, osteopathy, massages ...).

Category 2: As 1 + nontraditional methods (homeopathy, acupuncture, Spiritual healing ...) + Application of naturopathy.

Category 3: As 2 + support for self-help and for self-healing and to assume the responsibility; in parallel.

Category 4: No more action is needed because therapy is completed.

Note: With the progression of internal growth, external aids (medicines and other applications) are always less. In addition, the focus of energetic influence (treatment, application or therapy) is shifting more and more in the direction of higher energy levels. This means, with the progression of inner growth less and less orthodox medicine is required, while the alternative healing methods are preferred. At the same time the feeling of self-responsibility and self-empowerment is increasingly growing in order to can solve gradually the own problems, in whatever form they may look.

On the subject of spiritual healing and healers.

Spiritual healing, which is carried out externally, is to be interpreted on my viewpoint in a way, that the 'healer' serves only as a living catalyst, which brings in motion the healing process in the other. Only if the 'healer' conveys to his client his true function as a catalyst, he is really helping his client to find whose future salvation in himself. So, the healer gives to understand the client that his aid only is or was an aid to whose self-help or self-healing.

Also therapist, naturopath or doctor can be construed as 'healer' if acting in a harmonious way at any energetic level. Of course, everyone has just by its existence an energetic influence, because everyone is living energy. However, our influence may favor, depending on our intention and/or our spiritual state, either the course of a particular recovery or the course of a particular disease in the others, if the others are receptive to our influence in any form.

Now, the healer (= alive healing catalyst) can act on different planes, wherein the spiritual level is the most effective level of healing. **If the healer is capable of acting on the soul level, spontaneous healings may occur.** On the lower levels, the cure will be more of a temporal process and not as strong or powerful as at soul level. It may even be that the healing process is barely noticeable if it is influenced on the lower levels. The aim of every healer, therapist or life consultant should be, to bring his client to take advantage of external support only temporary in order to become gradually more independent through more intrinsic activity.

Soul plan and state of spirit (frame of mind).

Nothing can happen, if our state of spirit or our soul-plan does not allow it. It is evident, that the law of cause and effect can never be repealed. Therefore all healings have always to do with the state of mind and the soul plan of the respective participants. It should even be speculated that the soul plan is hierarchically above the mental condition, see "hidden causes, underlying causes" in part B.

If someone could be taken away a problem, such as a disease symptom, without he is able to see a reason to change his life accordingly, then this would not be in accordance with his soul plan. Thus, the problem solution (e.g. certain cure) will not be possible without a certain learning effect.

On the subject of state of spirit (frame of mind), we can ask the following questions: "How much confidence do we have in our life, in ourselves and in our inner guidance? What faith and confidence can we have that it happens to us only in such a way that it conforms always to our inner convictions, beliefs, fears, visions and the like? How well we succeed in finding enough time for relaxation, peace and quiet in our daily lives?" See "physiological aspect of the consideration of diseases" in part B.

Well, someone, who can act on soul level, knows exactly what he has to do on the others. He will act on the others only in such a way that it conforms always to their soul-plan, that it serves best their development and that he himself does not suffer any disadvantage. He knows that abuse of power could lead to the loss of the own power.

The one who can act only on the lower levels has more likely to follow his intuition. He will not be entirely free of self-interest and/or selfish motives. Because the ego, considered neutrally and without assessment, will be in the game for varying degrees, the therapeutic projects will be crowned with fluctuating success or not always successful or noticeable. Here it is, that both concerned parties have still to learn ("healer" like client). Anyway, those are to be found who are attracted to each other in accordance with the Law of Attraction. That means, clients and healers are always meeting in accordance with certain points of contact (study topics) that are somehow common or similar to each other.

Merger of several persons who give assistance.

It could prove to be very useful to provide an address for covering as many as possible areas, similar to a therapeutic or health center. This center should be geared at best that all disciplines are covered to make possible this synergy. This means that this requires a cooperation of visionaries, economists, agronomists (provision of healthy food), chefs (adequate preparation of food), doctors, Vision trainers, personal trainers, medical practitioners, naturopaths, various therapists (wellness, physiotherapy, psychotherapy, ...) and (Spirit-) healers. The establishment of such a center can be carried out by stages, so as to achieve and optimize the mentioned synergy step by step.

It is the time of mergers, of formation of groups, of networking, of mutual support and assistance, of mutual helping-together, of mutual healing, of Each Other and of coexistence. It is the time to give actively evidence that we are bound together in spirit. It is the time that healings and other miracles widely happen, that enthusiasm will be aroused as well as the memory of our all spiritual connectedness.

B: Possible causes of disease symptoms and symptomatology of the new time.

Physiological aspect of the consideration of diseases.

In nature, we can observe a certain relationship between tension (stress; be hunted by the enemy ...) and relaxation (to be left alone, to be protected, by playing ...). An animal that is being chased by another animal, is temporarily in the tension until it has found shelter. In shelter or if no enemy is near, it can recover and relax again.

If in nature the state of the tension takes the least time and if the state of relaxation is maintaining the greatest part of time then there is a balanced healthy relationship. In this day and age it can be observed in humans that the stress state occupies a large part of the time. We must protect ourselves constantly against something, must be on the alert and we take only a little time for reflection or for Muse. How often do we chase after different activities, those or other sensations, those or other adventures? Even if we want to relax, our thoughts revolve constantly about things/ topics that are causing problems, that worry, hinder or annoy us that we really cannot relax. How often we worry about things that happen quite differently and we can observe again and again that we have wasted a considerable time with it?

At the cellular level, it is to observe that the body cells are either in growth state or in protection state. Stress, anxiety, fear, anger, and the like bring the cells in the protection state. In this state, they cannot grow and therefore not regenerate. But to regeneration they need relaxation. This makes it clear that continuous stress, a lot of trouble, constant effort and/or constant worry suppress the immune system. Such a state thus is largely responsible for an unhealthy condition of the body. These attitudes have ultimately to do with the lack of inner confidence. For as long as our confidence is not great enough in ourselves, we would by overexertion, bustle, battle, defense, stress, anger and the like try to compensate that what we would achieve in confidence with ease.

Just as a state of relaxation outweighs in nature, it is to aim to come into a relaxed state in daily life - apart from rare and short-lived exceptions -, that our body can kept in a healthy condition. The lack of confidence shifts the natural relationship between tension and relaxation in an unfavorable area that it can cause problems to the body or bodily feeling. In other words, an unnatural relationship between tension and relaxation can make noticeable phenomena which are commonly understood as a disease. Now, we have a first approach in the understanding of disease symptoms.

Hidden causes/ underlying causes.

Even people who like to keep for positive thinking people are often confronted with illnesses and other problems. What could be wrong? I think that on the one hand every person is different in spiritual constitution and has a different life plan on the other hand. This plan can contain self-concepts, tasks or functions that can be so different that we can discuss only few examples.

A man perhaps has taken on the task in this life to eke out an existence as Crippled to iron out an act that he has committed once in a previous life and that do sorry to him, in other words, he decided to punish himself or at least to want to know also the side of a victim. It could also be that he wants by his crippled state to trick two soul mates, who are now his earthly father and his earthly mother, into becoming compassionate, that their petrified heart may soften a bit more.

Or, the soul of a child has decided to go early from this world - perhaps in the earthly sense too early. For instance, the then 16-year-old daughter of an acquaintance (a friend of mine) came to dead. This daughter had intuitively already known, that she would die soon, and told it her family. Only she did not know how she would die. This acquaintance is sometimes in contact with the spiritual world and also in contact with her daughter from the beyond. Through meditation she learned of her daughter from the beyond, that she can help people a lot better about the afterlife than she would do it on earth as a human being if she would have continued her earthly life. In this respect it is or was because of the new tasks from higher view better to dwell no longer on earth. Therefore her relatively early death had for other reasons a deeper sense.

Of course, there are other aspects that we can consider. Before incarnating many of us have planned in a higher consciousness a specific task that we necessarily want to run in this life (soul plan). We also knew about the fact that in the limited state of consciousness we would run into the risk by certain things or situations to be dazzled and distracted. So we would not always do that, what we want to do from the innermost core. How differently as by creating diseases, hurdles, obstacles and the like, we can be dissuaded from the error path? However, these situations are not made at random chance, but are in such a form that they can be interpreted. They are like a warning light, which makes itself noticeable if something is wrong, on that this wrong path will be rectified (illness as guidance).

These few examples should show that it usually looks quite different from an earthly perspective as from the higher point of view, wherein the true state of affairs is usually in secret and that isn't accessible to us normally. The earthly viewpoint is deceptive and often leads us to respond incomprehensibly to this or that or not to judge lawfully. This is exactly, what is often the problem of dealing with problem situations of various kinds. Here, there is often a lack of deeper insights.

The Lost Son and the Lost Daughter.

According to my understanding, there was a time in which once we all were one Spirit and we were fully aware of our wholeness, holiness, integrity and grandeur. This was a sort of paradisiacal state. The idea to live up fully our individuality has led us into oblivion and into the dullness. We can imagine this in such a way that we had formed body to our liking and organized with him a masquerade. If the contours of the body is to be changed at will, means this that the one form has to die so that other form can be born. Since we are initially still aware of our true identity we had not really understood the death of the body as a death.

Now, over time the body as mask gradually became independent, because it got a life of its own, which has gradually led to forget our true self and therefore to forget that we are the authors of these masks. While the awareness of our spiritual identity was brought to the background the perception of the body was brought to the fore. So, the awareness of our spiritual identity went almost completely lost. As a result, the idea of individuation has led, inter alia, to conflicts, to injury and to confrontation with the death of the body, wherein now with its death the extinction of the self has been associated, so that the fear has been created.

In a certain way we are stepped out of the paradisiacal state, like the Lost Son, who wanted to make his own experiences - separated from the oneness. His experiences were, inter alia, also associated with much pain, false starts and dead ends. But at some point these pains and the longing for his homeland have become so large that he had decided to return back.

We are now at the point where we have done enough experience in life of separateness, where at the same time many things came to ahead (intensified in a way) that it is hardly bearable for many people. We are virtually at a turning point with the words: **"This far and no further"**. The pain has now been achieved on many, so now those are willing to give up the old patterns, old behaviors and ways of thinking. Now we are also applicable to look a little more behind the scenes of things that we are really able to recognize that only trust (in the inner guide as well as in a good outcome of all things), forgiveness, hope, charity and love are our salvation, which means, that these elements help us to find the way home.

Without pain we would not question things, we would not speculate on the meaning of our lives, we would not feel any motivation of rethinking. Without pain our hearts could hardly be softened and we would feel no incentive to go new paths. To that extent, the pain has the function of shaking up, and nothing is so bad that it did not contain something positive.

In my view we consider hardships, problems and diseases mostly as something too bad or negative. In reality, they are there to be averted, solved and resolved. Because they do not simply arise or emerge out of the blue because of alleged injustices in the world, but they have the cause in our spirit. They are signs or guidance that give us direction. As such, they are indeed fortunate for us.

All things in the material world that exist together in interaction, are all manifestations that point to a complex state of spirit. And just this is the cause of the interaction of these things. So, everything that is happening in our lives on the material plane, does have the cause in our spirit. **The exterior is a pure effect and refers to our thoughts, feelings, our inner beliefs, visions, concepts and fears.** Because it refers to our spirit, it has a symbolic character. Therefore disease symptoms serve as interpretable warning signals. Insofar, characters are constantly sent to us according to our state of mind that accurately reflect our state of spirit.

For example, if a serious decision is pending and we just feel headache in this difficult situation, it has something to tell us. Perhaps the time for a decision is not the right. The head is the area of mind. In case that we are in conflict, then this can cause us headaches downright. Let us therefore check our plan and let us try to look at our current situation in a different light!

The type of accident can help us in our life. If we, for example, are skidded by car, we may have come figuratively also skidding in life. Even if we have entered into a shit, this has something to tell us. This may be a sign that we are not very attentive now. This character might warn us not to take the next step unpremeditated. Who is repeatedly confronted with bone fractures, should consider whether he should give up his hard and inflexible way, to try it more with softness and flexibility. Who always reacts to unpleasant situations with rigor or wishes for the impossible, wears down himself. He's getting more and more brittle, which, inter alia, shows by means of brittle bones. **We see, behind such accidents or situations it could be warnings for protecting us from an even bigger accident or disaster.**

The inner and outer (im-)balance.

Because we as immortal spirit are over matter, we have the power to bring to disappear every disease. Illness, injury and death are not really existent. They are only based on a belief that our body is our true identity and we are vulnerable and mortal in consequence. Accordingly, we believe that we have to protect our bodies or to have no reason for relaxation, peace, carelessness, joy, love, fun and games in this or that situation.

Illness or other regrettable circumstances are indications that the perfect confidence in ourselves and in the world is lacking and that we do not follow our soul plan. This is evident in the daily life practice therein that we dwell too often and for too long in a state of tension and stress, which lets manifest the unintended symptoms. The obstacle to enjoy life or to have the courage to do exactly what we would inwardly prefer to do, is based on an attitude that does not correspond to our true nature. These barrier keeps our body cells in protection feature, what favors the disease of the body.

The transformation.

Injuries or experiences from previous incarnations are not really forgotten. They are hidden and deeply rooted in us. Because they are constantly present as vibrating information, they emboss in any form our mental attitude: Dislikes for this, fears for that, barriers to this, an inferiority complex in this or that area, and so on, that we cannot really bring in connection with our behavior of our today's earthly existence. Some might have an aversion to the church, even though they see no real reason for this aversion, which could be justified by the fact that they were executed in a previous life as a heretic by the Inquisition. The others have a tight-feeling if a chain is placed around their neck, which could be justified by the fact that they were strangled once in a previous life. I myself had about 2-3 weeks pain in the upper body, as if I had been pierced by several daggers. This pain came out of the blue (without injury), but disappeared again as if by magic.

We live in a time in which external energies (energy of the Photon Belt, in which our solar system penetrates more and more; other cosmic energies) **and internal energies** (Kundalini energy of the people, higher dimensional energies) **flow**

through us, whether that we work with any energy or we are simply receptive to it. These energies lead to the dissolution of energy blockades, which let reawaken old thought and behavior patterns as well as memories of past injuries in an attenuated form that they can disappear forever.

If symptoms occur out of the blue, this could mean that the corresponding internal settings/beliefs (unpurified past) are now ready to be transferred into the light, to speak, to be rethought, so that we gradually come into a state of mind that corresponds to God's nature. It is to say, that God's nature is also our all nature.

In the course of this harmonization the unpurified past will be purified as if by magic, in which the pain of old injuries rise briefly again in weakened form and without real damage, so that it can be lighted from new. Only then, if in this new lighting we can bring the former wrong thinking and feeling back in the right light, we can let go of it. Then the old disharmonious seeming information will be converted (transformed) into a new harmonious seeming information what brings us in a (more) relaxed mindset and brings the cells of our body in the growth state or may hold them in this state.

Categorization of disease symptoms.

Now we have addressed a wide range of possible causes of disease symptoms, which all have their origin in the spirit. Disease symptoms may be due to self-concepts that either have something to do with sacrifice or atonement (self-punishment): **This may be symptoms or pains of the first kind.** Other symptoms or pains may have to do with the fact that they want to put us on the path to our true happiness (**symptoms or pains of the second kind**). Over the pain the symptoms want to divert us from a path which, if we were to continue it in the same manner, would not lead us to our true happiness or would not let satisfy our longings.

In other words. Over the pain we are forced repeatedly to pause, that we are able to think or feel about ourselves and about the world to get into a mental attitude (mindset) that can evoke our spiritual consciousness and that can bring us at the end into the state of spiritual awareness. In state of spiritual awareness we would have found true fulfillment and therefore we will do nothing that would injure our body or would inflict pain on us or the other. As seen, the symptom or pain of the second type may be a useful warning sign, which will bring us on the way to ourselves and which will remind us that we have gone really astray.

Once we have progressed on our journey of self-discovery so far that generally we are very relaxed, very self-conscious and with great confidence to the day's work and/or to the future, we perhaps will be primarily confronted only with **symptoms or pains of the third kind.** These are "old-known" pains, which emerge again in a weakened form (out of the blue) by action of inner energies (Kundalini energy, higher dimensional energies) and external energies (e.g. cosmic energies), then to be dissolved (transformed) forever. Nevertheless, it is to make clear that we can be faced on the path to self-discovery with symptoms that may have to do with adapting difficulties of our bodies to the new energies. This can e.g. happen if we are tempted to want to accelerate our development process.

Symptoms or pains of the fourth kind (adapting difficulties of the body). We live in a time in which themes of self-discovery, self-healing, self-realization and self-development are processed intensively. A corollary is that we are reinforced faced with different energies (subtle energies, higher dimensional energies, cosmic energies and so on). These energies are unaccustomed for our bodies.

Then, if these unfamiliar energies start pouring too much or too fast into our energy body system, there may be certain difficulties in adjusting and adapting of our body. Here we have then to do with symptoms of the 4th kind, wherein the Kundalini energy of man may be also in a considerable degree at work here. It must be said that this energy is in every human being. It is a subtle energy that quasi has rested or slept for most people in the past and thereby has been entirely unnoticeable. In a time of increased exposure of energy and the self-development this energy will be awoken in man in a strengthened way: in the one more in the other less.

Regardless of the strength of the awakening, the Kundalini energy has the task to flow through all the energy pathways of our energy body system. By its flow it solves gradually all possible energy blockades and lets the Aura more and more unfold. At the same time this energy harmonizes the aura centers (chakras, which are like transmitting and receiving antennas) one after the other, so that the aura will become more and more receptive to higher dimensional energies. So, the Kundalini ensures that internal higher dimensional energies can flow in and can be incorporated in the aura system. This contributes to the overall harmonization of the energy body system and thus to the energy blockade solution at all possible levels. About this way our mind gets clearance. Once all energy blockades are dissolved, our mind can be connected along the main power canal over the Crown Chakra with the cosmic consciousness, so as to cancel the limits of mind. **Thus, the Kundalini energy is something like a pioneer for the liberation of our mind.**

Now it may be that the soul of a person feels a great urge to advance the liberation of the mind. If the mind of this person (ego), however, has refused to work on his liberation, it may now be that the soul abuts that exemption by creating situations that greater amounts of Kundalini energy will be released in the body. If the man has not ensured in advance to prepare his energy body system for this energy, it may be that this Kundalini awakening now causes greater difficulties. It may also be that large amounts of Kundalini could be released, in case that you are strongly drugged, by making exaggerated meditation exercises or even by deliberately making exercises for Kundalini release.

If the energy body system is not prepared for a particular strength of Kundalini release, there may be adapting and adjusting difficulties of our body,

<u>that can strongly strain the body:</u> flashes of light, then chills, hearing voices, from on top of the world to in the depths of despair by the one moment to the next, similar symptoms of schizophrenia, and so on. Such people suddenly can be very highly energy charged and can sometimes be very unbearable. It may also be that such people suddenly (for some moments) are mentally deranged and suffer from a relatively large loss of reality. It may also happen that momentarily the vertebrae of the spine are shifting or the organs in the body are shifting, that the Kundalini energy paves its way pop-like or explosively and that the whole body energy system can be messed up. This can go so far that the functions of the body are completely muddled up (death-like conditions) for a short time, which may be associated simultaneously with extracorporeal experiences. Man can so come to a limit between "death" and life over a certain period. How this process will run, will here be unpredictable. Here trust is then truly necessary in the highest degree.

In case, that such extreme symptoms emerge, it is very important that you do not get panic and you do not try to do or to let do things too quickly, that could aggravate the situation even more. For such people it is very important that emotional support is provided for them, that great patience is applied to them that you care about them, but also that them is given the peace (silence, rest) that they need.

For a certain time, I took in charge of a young woman who had withdrawal symptoms of psychotropic drugs as well as a Kundalini crisis. Experience with this woman showed that one couldn't assign in the respective moments, whether such extreme conditions were based on the withdrawal effects or of Kundalini crisis. It should be well known that even with withdrawal symptoms people can come to the limit between life and "death" as it is also possible at a Kundalini crisis.

I speak of phenomena, for which a diagnosis in the classical sense is not always possible or where things are at play that are so far largely unknown in classical medicine. If such phenomena are degenerating, there is no silver bullet and no guarantee of anything, no matter at what measures we let us tempt. Whether we treat this symptoms or not, it can go either way out.

The use of medication such as psychotropic drugs should be considered as a last resort and in any case carried out with caution here. If possible, friends, acquaintances or family members should take in charge such a person in his usual familiar environment as long as he has made a recovery. Of course, situationally doctors or therapists can be consulted. However, the path to psychiatry should be considered as a last resort.

Although I pointed out possible extreme cases, it should be made clear that these cases are not the rule and that they are among the really few exceptions. But they are accumulating nowadays to my finding (due to personal reports) more and more. In general, the Kundalini experiences can be mastered relatively well, they are anyway to come to liberation of the mind.

It is really amazing that in spite of the above-described extreme conditions (in the cases known to me) no real harm has arisen to the body. That is why it is so helpful to know about the phenomena associated with the Kundalini energy or other Light Body or transformation processes. With this knowledge it can be removed the breeding ground for certain fears. Because with fear, we run slightly risk to do things that could aggravate the situation even more. **While we have normally to do nothing more than to let happen and to endure, it is natural to explore in extreme cases how far we place our lives in God's hands or/and in the hands of doctors and therapists.**

To my experience with the Kundalini energy see: http://www.amazon.com/Personal-experience-Kundalini-spiritual-backgrounds-ebook/dp/B01BJ2T404/ref=sr_1_1?s=digital-text&ie=UTF8&qid=1456784648&sr=1-1

Note. In understanding of disease symptoms the German New Medicine® is likely to be very enlightening (http://www.newmedicine.ca/). This medicine was developed by Ryke Geerd Hamer and is based on Five Biological Laws. According to this medicine all disease symptoms would run after these 5 biological laws. The emergence and disappearance of symptoms are considered each as part of a typically biphasic "Meaningful Special Biological Program" (MSBP). After Hamer the trigger of each so-called symptoms is always a biological conflict, a highly dramatic shock experience, the so-called DHS (Dirk-Hamer-Syndrome).

As I understand, the German New Medicine® provides a very good approach in the understanding of such disease symptoms, which result in conjunction with concrete conflict situations. Nevertheless, I think that this medicine cannot explain or cover all symptoms. The symptoms that result from the "Meaningful Special Biological

Program" (MSBP), I would regard as symptoms of the second kind.

Summary of part B.

Severe symptoms that traditional medicine regards as incurable or that have something to do with deformities, may be caused, inter alia, by the aforementioned self-concepts and self-punishments, which in certain circumstances could be maintained over more than one incarnation. This of course depends on how long the soul of the respective person decides to maintain such a self-concept.

Moderate to heavy symptoms might already be a certain shaking up (waking up) to lead us to the right path due to our soul plan. Here, the soul has perhaps already reached a higher maturity to seek now primarily salvation as the goal (illness as way). This soul perhaps makes use of pains or problems only from the motivation to bring us back from our self-destructive path. For this we can also count strokes of fate that tempt us to come to a different way or different Living.

The desirable (new) Living will have something to do with trust, letting go, love, understanding, compassion, joy, fun and games.

Those who have already gained more confidence in their life and follow more their intuition, will be faced with symptoms and problems that are more of the third kind, sometimes of the 4th kind. This means, symptoms now will almost exclusively emerge due to old hidden injuries in weakened form in order then to disappear forever.

Of course, spiritually advanced people will also stumble sometimes, because they too are still trying to be guided by things that they let derail. This also means that some minor injuries or accidents or illnesses can occur that we, on the other hand, can easily iron out or heal quickly. These then serve as signs about with the words: *"Take it easy! Stop and come back to your center! Have faith and do everything with caution and with the help of your inner intuition ".*

The time of self-discovery, self-healing, self-realization and self-development let's get a little more back in touch with our divine nature. But this also goes hand in hand with the fact that we are confronted with different energies (subtle energies, higher dimensional energies, cosmic energies, inner energies) and that we are increasingly encouraged to learn how to deal with them. By this influence the higher dimensional energies are introduced into our energy body system. This in turn means that the so-called light body process causes at the lower levels of the energy body system a restructuring or redesign.

If this energy-effects take place too fast or too violent, it may be that we get adapting and adjustment difficulties of our bodies, which can manifest in the form of fatigue, exhaustion, or even in the form of physical ailments of varying amounts. These symptoms are concomitants of this adjustment difficulties due to the transformation or metamorphosis process that runs in the course of this self-discovery by itself.

Concomitants may also exist in various therapeutic applications such as acupuncture, acupressure, massage, physiotherapy and other therapies as well as spiritual healing, because it generally can lead to energy blockades resolutions here. At this point, it should again be emphasized that the symptoms of the 3rd and 4th kind are phenomena that cannot be really diagnosed in conventional medical sense. Those symptoms can be severe at times, but usually they do not damage our bodies and disappear relatively quickly. That is, they are characterized in particular by the fact that they emerge out of the blue and disappear relatively quickly without requiring to be treated. The symptoms, with whom I personally made experience and which I would place in the category 3 or 4, lasted up to 4 weeks, but mostly disappeared after a few days or hours. In order that these symptoms do not occur so much in extent, it is useful in energy work to deal wisely with the higher dimensional energies and always to ground yourself what can be achieved, inter alia, with the so-called 4-body grounding (earthing).

Our ultimate goal is the liberation of our mind. The closer we go to this destination, with the more powerful energies we have to do and the greater is the challenge to learn to deal masterfully with these energies, so that it serves best our spiritual development. In this sense, I wish us all a good hand in our decisions for all our activities and a wise recognition for what may lie ahead for us in the new time.

C: Suggestion for finding our own Honor Codex.

We are accustomed to act in accordance to standards, guidelines, commandments, ordinances and laws, perhaps without having questioned whether these requirements are still the right means for a free cooperation. Certainly these requirements have been justified so far in order to ensure a certain order among men. But I think from a certain maturity of people it might be required to move gradually away from the fixed attitudes, in order to trust more and more our own feelings, the inner wisdom and inner impulses. Because our inner wisdom knows the true principles of a free and carefree existence, we also will, if we let ourselves be guided by it, be able to achieve such a free existence.

Since I'm working extensively with the theme healing and I see myself partially in the function as a bioenergy therapist, I was looking, inter alia, for a Codex for doctors, therapists and other acting people in medical system, which is likely to help each other to achieve spiritual independence and to let unfold all our spiritual potential. But we can only reach this independence if everyone of us takes for himself his own Codex, in which function we want to see us in this existence (as a doctor, therapist, teacher, educator, client, patient, student, seeker ...). Of course each free being that we all are, has to find out, according to which Codex he would align his life.

In view of the finding of the own Codex there were or are a lot of good suggestions/ approaches such as Immanuel Kant's categorical imperative, the Hippocratic Oath, Declaration of Geneva (Physician's Oath), therapist-Codex (by Peter Orban), Codex Alimentarius, Codex Medicamentarius and the like. However, anyone has to find out his own Codex or with what suggestions he may come in resonance best.

As we learned, the deeper meaning of the term "medicament" points to the fact that in every being resides an inner healer (the real medicament), who's really able to heal. This healer has true wisdom that we can make ourselves available by calling over (by invoking) or/and by connecting with it.

Now, the following points should be seen under this background, which can, in my view, help us mutually to achieve the spiritual independence. In other words, if I was even in the function as a doctor, therapist or as a person who acts in the medical system in another way, I would match the following listed topics points:

1. **The doctor/ therapist aims for a treatment/ application/ therapy to make the patient/ client independent of himself.** Say he provides primarily to help people to help themselves and tries everything to reveal the causes of the symptoms of his patients/ clients to mobilize the self-healing powers and to strengthen their self-confidence. This means that the doctor/ therapist examines together with the patients/ clients for the causes of their symptoms, so that those can recognize them. The doctor/ therapist gives the patients/ clients ideally the feeling that the solution to their problem is in themselves, saying that they can solve their problem themselves.

2. **Medicament in pharmaceutical sense and/or applications or treatments, whatsoever, should always be viewed as a temporary aid until the client/ patient has recognized the real cause of his symptoms.** Medicaments in pharmaceutical sense or particular applications or treatments cannot really heal. They can relieve symptoms at most. Real symptom resolution is only possible by the cause solution. If only symptom treatment is carried out - without

cause solution - a symptom displacement is achieved with high probability, which is no real cure. Then it is launched a vicious spiral. This spiral can only be broken by a cause solution.

3. **The message of diagnoses to the patient/ client conveys to him the feeling that he is really ill, instead the understanding that there is a cause for his symptoms, which can be changed by himself.** The feeling of being ill or to have a particular disease, is a certain feeling of helplessness. It gives him at the same time the feeling to be dependent on "the man/ woman in the white coat", which prevents man to go into self-responsibility. By contrast, the knowledge that there is a cause for each symptom, which is to be sought in everyone, leads to a behavior, that the man himself lends a hand to identify the causes. In this way he will be motivated to go into the self-responsibility.

4. **In the healing/ recovery of the patient/ client the doctor/ therapist can hold the following key features:**
   - In the function of a catalyst he sets virtually in motion a self-healing in the patient/ client what is possible about the building of trust, by establishing of mutual sympathy, by

encouragement and/or by any other energetic action, as over a certain healing technique.

- He helps the patient/ client to get access to the inner wisdom/ knowledge that he's able to detect the cause of his symptoms/ problems.
- He prescribes measures to alleviate the symptoms or even performs them with the background to encourage the client/ patient at the same time to search for the real causes of his symptoms.
- The measures for symptoms such as bone fractures are of course arranged or carried out in a way that the self-healing forces can act in an optimal way. Here is to be given an understanding to the patient/ client that such a measure (for example to put an arm in plaster) has no healing properties in itself, but that the actual healing takes place in himself.
- When deciding which measures have to be considered for symptom alleviating the physician/ therapist has to find out for which measure the client/ patient can win confidence or has most trust. So, the responsibility is no more passed solely on the doctor/ therapist but is also transferred to the patient/ client.

5. **It is to aim for a synergy of all disciplines in medical system.** This synergy depends on the level of knowledge of physician and therapist on the one hand and on the understanding of the patient/ client on the other. If a physician or therapist feels that he's not competent enough in a particular issue or he has some doubts about his treatment, it goes without saying, that an interdisciplinary exchange is wanted. If different treatment methods come in question it should be chosen such a treatment for which the patient/ client can get the most confidence.

6. **The basic idea of synergy is that any form of therapy, treatment or use in principle has its special place**, if an implementation is carefully and professionally done wherein it is to work out together with the patient/ client which therapy, treatment or application has the best chance of success in relieving symptoms. This requires that the practitioners of the different areas in medical system are in an interconnected exchange at eye level and that they seek together for the best solution according to their level of knowledge. In the following points 7 and 8 it will be discussed, how the best solution can be found.

7. **Each health center should try to ask in service as wide a range of aid workers in accordance with the previous points**, so to offer in this way a complementary medicine and to advance the mentioned synergy. This means that this requires a cooperation of visionaries, economists, agronomists (provision of healthy food), chefs (adequate preparation of food), doctors, Vision trainers, personal trainers, medical practitioners, naturopaths, various therapists (wellness, physiotherapy, psychotherapy, ...) and (Spirit) healers. The establishment of such a center can be done in stages, so as to achieve and optimize step by step the mentioned synergy.

8. **Despite complexity it is to strive a simplicity.** The holistic approach of the American-Israeli medical sociologist Aaron Antonovsky, which brings in supplementary to each other the Pathogenesis and the so called **Salutogenesis** as a concept, goes certainly in the right direction: see: http://www.bzga.de/botmed_60606000.html. **Quick note on this subject:** *Aaron Antonovsky criticizes a purely pathogenetic-curative Viewing manner and provides in addition to it a salutogenetic perspective which primarily asks*

why people stay healthy, instead only to ask for disease causes and risk factors.

Likewise, the concept of Ryke Geerd Hamer (German New Medicine®) is, in my view, very revealing, see: http://www.newmedicine.ca/. Nevertheless it should be considered that each person is unique and has individual topics, problems, settings and the like. So, if we invoke the inner wisdom of each person, everything will be simplified in an optimal way (Tags: to follow the plan of life, to listen to the inner guide, to accept the life issue, to satisfy the inner longings and impulses, to investigate the true divine nature, ...).

9. **It is considered that the ultimate goal of every human being is to follow his true calling, vocation and mission.** The man who has reached this achievable goal - and every man can work toward this goal, if he is capable of independent thinking - can be regarded as safe and free from fear.

10. **According to this view any situation, where a person is located, corresponds exactly to his individual (un-)consciousness.** The path is virtually from the unconsciousness (state in which a person is not (yet) aware of his true

divinity) to the conscious awareness (state in which the human being is fully aware of his true divinity). The man who is fully aware of his true divinity can follow his true divine nature, can always satisfy his inner desires/ impulses, is free from fear and can always pursue his day's work in a relaxed way. The formation of disease symptoms for such a person does not make sense anymore, because he is now in perfect harmony with himself and the world. The formation of such symptoms may primarily, if not exclusively, be regarded as warning signs to bring us to such path which leads us to our true fulfillment, freedom, satisfaction, happiness and recollection of who we are in reality.

11. **Therapist and doctor can understand themselves as the patient/ client in the higher sense, provided that they are not (yet) aware of their divinity.** As long as they are not aware of this, they are even not free of problems, disease symptoms and conflicts. Only such an interaction between therapists/ doctors and clients/ patients, by which an inner connection with their counterparts is achieved to make the voice of the inner wisdom of each concerned parties be heard, leads to psycho-energetic

harmonic resonance. This harmonic resonance in turn can cause that healing and/ or a recollection of who we are can take place. Of course, from this resonance patients/ clients as well as therapists/ doctors benefit.

12. **In terms of a real healing, it's not so very crucial which concrete measure, therapy or treatment is prescribed or carried out. In this respect the generation and increasing of resonance in the energy body system is much more crucial.** So, what is relevant is the intention of finding lovingly common ways that sends all concerned parties into the autonomy and independence under appeal to the inner healer or inner wisdom. If therapists and physicians are superfluous in the end for the client/ patient, they are at the same time free. Someone, who wants completely to be independent and free, can never achieve this, if he makes others dependent of himself (see point 1). The absence or/ and the wavering or not reproducibility of healing effects is probably due to the fact that it does not always come to a harmonious resonance between doctor/ therapist and patient/ client or between patient/ client and

his situation. Reasons that a resonance cannot be established, may be, for example:

- The giving of diagnoses scares patient/ client (point 3)
- There exists a distrust or antipathy ratio between doctor/ therapist and patent/ client or it comes to such a ratio
- The uncomfortable feeling in patient/ client couldn't be converted in a trusting feeling.

Of course, it may also be that a certain cure then does not take place if it's not consistent with the mental condition or with the soul plan of the help-seeker, so, if the help-seeker would not change his life concept at a possible cure.

13. **Finally, the problems of the patients/ clients can't be seen isolated from the problems of the doctor/ therapist.** Such a conjuncture (meeting) of both sides has finally mutually chance of healing, of redemption, of the development of spiritual potential and of the complete recollection of what we really are.

In regard to cause solution. Perhaps it's not always so important to know what exactly the causes of our problems are. Often, it is sufficient by *simply to know that some symptoms are part of an overall purification process that wants to lead us more and more to our true nature. Other symptoms or problems will be based on our own life concepts, which are not in consistence with our divine nature. **If we bring, in turn, our life in accordance with our true nature, then a great number of symptoms or problems - if not all - will disappear.** Therefore, it is usually better to reflect on our true nature (medi[cament]um) and then to try to act according to it, instead to try to identify each cause of anything. **Again:** Usually it is mostly better, to let bring by simply old behavior and thinking patterns behind us and just to try to live our life according to our true divine nature and to the inner impulses. So, it is mostly better just to live, instead of constantly wasting the time with brooding, pondering and turning problems over in one's mind!!*

The basic idea of this codex can be applied on any other life areas such as school, education and partnerships, because it is always and everywhere the same spiritual principle. Your problem is not separate from my problem, no matter whether I am teacher or student, doctor or patient, therapist or client. In all cases, we enter into a relationship that always opens up the possibility of healing, of redemption, of the development of our spiritual potential up to the complete recollection of what we really are and that we all are one.

That we all are interconnected and that everything has to do with everything, is ultimately a quantum physical result. Because the whole is in every small particles from quantum physics perspective, everything is connected with everything else. Therefore, our problems cannot be seen separately from the problems of others. **So healing can only happen, if we transform in the interaction with the other the feeling of separation** ("I'm worth more than you; I know more than you; your problem is not my problem; I am above thee; ...") **into the feeling of "connectedness"**, that we are each other brothers and sisters, that in each of us is all potential for our salvation and our independence or/ and that we belong together and we go towards a common goal. This transformation, with which a loving, respectful and honor bringing attitude towards the others goes always hand in hand, can take place at all levels of life. Because this conversion is of harmonious nature it entails always solution of problems, salvation, healing and/or happiness.

In every man lives inner wisdom. Although it may be that it is (still) hidden in many of us, it waits that we help and support each other to make it usable for us until we become completely aware of it. Likewise in every man lives an inner healer, who just waits, to can be developed fully in us. So, a common goal could be, that we assist and support each other in getting (back) the awareness of our wholeness, our divinity and our all connectedness. And so, such a codex could be useful to remind us again and again to this common goal.

The one who wants to be really aware
of the responsibility of himself and his fellows,
should always ask, if in doubt,
according to which Codex he wants to act.

Summary and Outlook.

More and more people are aware of the influence of spiritual energies to the visible gross material plane through the invisible subtle levels, get therein more and more insight and perceive healing. They develop talents and gifts which they apply with increasing success to themselves and others. This results in new occupations in the medical system (field of bioenergetics, psycho-energetics and spiritual healing).

Especially in this day and age, where people are getting sicker, more dissatisfied and frail in the scale of classical medicine and where medicine, classical or alternatively, reaches its limits the market is crying out for new occupations. It reveals by itself a new market. This market is going to be known and to be established increasingly. Let us fill in this gap and seize the opportunity with some courage!!!

It should be understood by now that we in fact have solutions to our true liberation. This requires the overarching cooperation of all disciplines, not only in the medical system but also in the sciences. All these disciplines can serve as a springboard to our primordial knowledge or for connecting with our primal matrix (blueprint). But they can be such a springboard only then if they are not placed in counter-position to each other but brought together in one common synthesis.

The result of this synthesis will be that the connection to the great-matrix (blueprint) can be facilitated, which is accompanied by the liberation of man. In my view, with respect to that connection the Keshe Blueprint technology could provide a good means for such a relief (see source). Certainly some experiences are still to be collected to be able to get better aware of the greatness of that technology.

It is also conceivable that the door to the Blueprint can be opened by means of high potencies of homeopathy and other alternative medicines. Here it will be very decisive how pure the intentions of the corresponding therapists, medical practitioner, physician or spirit healer and of course of the help-seekers is and/ or whether this opening is destined in the soul plan of the help-seeker.

Nevertheless, any extern aids or means should always be considered as temporary. They themselves may be only a stepping stone to our true liberation. Because true freedom always means to be independent of others and of any outer things or extern aids. True liberation is thus always an internal process, which, inter alia, is manifested by means of the Kundalini process. **The Kundalini energy is expected to play a key role in our liberation process.** And since it is a body's own energy it has automatically to do with the inner liberation process. Otherwise it would not be what it is.

The ultimate goal of every human being should be the liberation of the mind. The closer we go to this destination, with the more powerful energies we have to do and the greater is the challenge to learn to deal masterfully with these energies, so that it serves best our spiritual development. In this sense, I wish us all a good hand in our decisions for all our activities and a wise recognition for what may lie ahead for us in the new time.

Literature and sources.

Chakra Handbook; Sharamon, Shalia & Baginski and Bodo J.
http://www.amazon.com/The-Chakra-Handbook-Shalila-Sharamon/dp/094152485X

Kundalini and the Chakras", Genevieve Lewis Paulson
http://www.amazon.com/Kundalini-Chakras-Evolution-Lifetime-Llewellyns/dp/0875425925

The Subtle Body; Cyndi Dale
http://www.amazon.de/The-Subtle-Body-Encyclopedia-Energetic/dp/1591796717

Epigenetics
http://www.whatisepigenetics.com/fundamentals/

The salutogenic model as a theory to guide health promotion, from Aaron Antonovsky
http://heapro.oxfordjournals.org/content/11/1/11.abstract

Ruprecht-Karls-Universität Heidelberg, Manchmal hilft auch eine Scheinoperation (pseudo-operation does help sometimes)
http://www.uni-heidelberg.de/presse/news04/2402auch.html

Germanic/German New Medicine®
http://www.newmedicine.ca/
Keshe foundation (blueprint)
http://beforeitsnews.com/alternative/2015/10/keshe-releases-free-energy-blueprints-live-3233928.html
http://www.keshefoundation.org/

My website
http://www.franzguenter-leicht.info

About my personal experience with the Kundalini energy
http://www.amazon.com/Personal-experience-Kundalini-spiritual-backgrounds-ebook/dp/B01BJ2T404/ref=sr_1_1?s=digital-text&ie=UTF8&qid=1456784648&sr=1-1